# Breast Cancer Survivor's Guide

## From Diagnosis to Recovery

Rossana Lewis

# TABLE OF CONTENT

# Chapter 1: Understanding Breast Cancer

## 1.1 What is breast Cancer

Breast cancer is a disease in which abnormal breast cells grow out of control and form tumors. If left unchecked, the tumors can spread throughout the body and become fatal.

Breast cancer cells begin inside the milk ducts and/or the milk-producing lobules of the breast. The earliest form (in situ) is not life-threatening. Cancer cells can spread into nearby breast tissue (invasion). This creates tumors that cause lumps or thickening.

Invasive cancers can spread to nearby lymph nodes or other organs (metastasize). Metastasis can be fatal.

## 1.2 Types of breast cancer

Breast cancer is categorized into types and subtypes so treatment can be tailored to be as effective as possible with the fewest possible side effects. Common types of breast cancer include:

- Invasive (infiltrating) ductal carcinoma (IDC): This cancer starts in your milk ducts and spreads to nearby breast tissue. It's the most common type of breast cancer in the United States.
- Lobular breast cancer: This breast cancer starts in the milk-producing glands (lobules) in your breast and often spreads to nearby breast tissue. It's the second most common breast cancer in the United States.

- Ductal carcinoma in situ (DCIS): Like IDC, this breast cancer starts in your milk ducts. The difference is DCIS doesn't spread beyond your milk ducts.

Less common breast cancer types include:

- Triple-negative breast cancer (TNBC): This invasive cancer is aggressive and spreads more quickly than other breast cancers.

- Inflammatory breast cancer (IBC): This rare, fast-growing cancer looks like a rash on your breast. IBC is rare in the United States.

- Paget's disease of the breast: This rare cancer affects the skin of your nipple and may look like a rash. Less than 4% of all breast cancers are Paget's disease of the breast.

For breast cancer subtypes,    the cancer is classified by receptor cell status. Receptors are protein molecules in or on cells' surfaces. They can attract or attach to certain substances in your blood, including hormones like estrogen and progesterone. Estrogen and progesterone help cancerous cells to grow. Finding out if cancerous cells have estrogen or progesterone receptors helps healthcare providers plan breast cancer treatment.

Subtypes include:

- ER-positive (ER+) breast cancers have estrogen receptors.
- PR-positive (PR+) breast cancers have progesterone receptors.
- HR-positive (HR+) breast cancers have estrogen and progesterone receptors.

- HR-negative (HR-) breast cancers don't have estrogen or progesterone receptors.

- HER2-positive (HER2+) breast cancers, which have higher than normal levels of the HER2 protein. This protein helps cancer cells to grow. About 15% to 20% of all breast cancers are HER2-positive.

## 1.3 Stages of Breast Cancer

The stage of your cancer is based on the size of the tumor and if it has spread to other areas.

There are five stages of breast cancer, including 0 (zero) through 4, written as 0, I, II, III, and IV. The higher the number, the more the cancer has spread. The cancer is staged when you are first diagnosed. If you have Stage II breast cancer and the cancer comes back and spreads to your bone, you will still have Stage II breast cancer with metastasis (spread) to the bones.

The stage of breast cancer is also described by the "TNM" system:

T: Tumor size (in centimeters)

N: Number of nearby lymph nodes with cancer

M: Whether the cancer has metastasized or spread to other organs of the body (0 = no spread, 1 = it has spread)

Stage 0: The disease is only in the ducts and lobules of the breast. It has not spread to the surrounding tissue. It is also called noninvasive cancer (Tis, N0, M0).

Stage I: The disease is invasive. Cancer cells are now in normal breast tissue. There are 2 types:

- Stage IA: The tumor is up to 2 centimeters (cm). It has not spread to the lymph nodes (T1, N0, M0).

- Stage IB: The tumor is in the breast and is less than 2 cm. Or the tumor is in the lymph nodes of the breast and there is no tumor in the breast tissue.

Stage II describes invasive breast cancer. There are 2 types:

- Stage IIA: A tumor may not be found in the breast, but cancer cells have spread to at least 1 to 3 lymph nodes. Or Stage IIA may show a 2 to 5 cm tumor in the breast with or without spread to the axillary lymph nodes.

- Stage IIB: The tumor is 2 to 5 cm and the disease has spread to 1 to 3 axillary lymph nodes. Or the tumor is larger than 5 cm but has not spread to the axillary lymph nodes.

Stage III describes invasive breast cancer. There are 3 types:

- Stage IIIA: The tumor is in the breast and any size or no tumor is found in the breast but is in the lymph nodes. The disease has spread to more than 4 lymph nodes in the breast or axilla. It has not spread to other parts of the body.

- Stage IIIB: The tumor may be any size and the disease has spread to the chest wall. It may cause swelling of the breast and may be in up to 9 lymph nodes. Inflammatory breast cancer is considered Stage IIIB.

- Stage IIIC: There may be no sign of cancer in the breast or a tumor may be any size and may have spread to the chest wall or breast skin. The disease has spread to 10 or more axillary lymph nodes, or nodes above or below the collarbone or breastbone.

Stage IV (metastatic): The tumor can be any size and the disease has spread to other organs and tissues, such as the bones, lungs, brain, liver, distant lymph nodes, or chest wall (any T, any N, M1).

## 1.4 Risk Factors and Prevention

A risk factor is anything that increases a person's chance of developing cancer. Although risk factors often influence the development of cancer, most do not directly cause cancer. Some people with several risk factors never develop cancer, while others with no known risk factors do. Knowing your risk factors and talking about them with your doctor may help you make more informed lifestyle and health care choices.

Most breast cancers are sporadic, meaning they develop from damage to a person's genes that occurs by chance after they are born. Sporadic breast cancer means there is no risk of the person passing the gene on to their children. The underlying cause of sporadic breast cancer is a combination of internal, or hormonal, exposures; lifestyle factors; environmental factors; and normal physiology, such as DNA replication.

Inherited breast cancers are less common, making up about 10% of cancers. Inherited breast cancer occurs when gene changes, called mutations or alterations, are passed down within a family from parent to child. Many of those mutations are in tumor suppressor genes, such as BRCA1, BRCA2, and PALB2. These genes normally keep cells from growing out of control and turning into cancer. But when these cells have a mutation, it can cause them to grow out of control.

When considering your breast cancer risk, it is important to remember that a high majority of people who develop breast cancer have no obvious risk factors and no strong family history of breast cancer. Multiple risk factors influence the development of breast cancer. This means that all people need to be aware of changes in their breasts. They also need to talk with their doctor about recommendations for receiving regular breast examinations by a doctor as well as mammograms. A mammogram is an x-ray of the breast that can often find a tumor that is too small to be felt.

The following factors may raise a person's risk of developing breast cancer:

Age: The risk of developing breast cancer increases with age, with most cancers developing after age 50. The median age for developing breast cancer is 63.

Personal history of breast cancer: A woman who has had breast cancer in 1 breast has a higher risk of developing a new cancer in the other breast.

Family history of breast cancer: Breast cancer may run in the family in any of these situations:

- 1 or more women are diagnosed with breast cancer at age 45 or younger
- 1 or more women are diagnosed with breast cancer before age 50 with an additional family history of cancer, such as ovarian cancer, metastatic prostate cancer, and pancreatic cancer.
- There are breast and/or ovarian cancers in multiple generations on 1 side of the family, such as having both a grandmother and an aunt on the father's side of the family who were both diagnosed with 1 of these cancers.
- A woman in the family is diagnosed with a second breast cancer in the same or the other breast or has both breast and ovarian cancer.
- A relative is diagnosed with male breast cancer

Inherited risk/genetic predisposition: There are several inherited genetic mutations linked with an increased risk of breast cancer, as well as other types of cancer. BRCA1 or BRCA2 are the most common known genes linked to breast cancer. Mutations in these genes are linked to an increased risk of breast and ovarian cancers, as well as other types of cancer. Male breast cancer, as well as the risk for prostate cancer and other cancers, is also increased if there is a mutation in 1 of these genes. Learn more about hereditary breast and ovarian cancer in a more detailed guide on this website.

Other gene mutations or hereditary conditions can increase a person's risk of breast cancer. They are far less common than BRCA1 or

BRCA2, and they do not increase the risk of breast cancer as much.

Early menstruation and late menopause: If menstruation began before ages 11 or 12 or menopause began after age 55, there is a somewhat higher risk of breast cancer. This is because the breast cells have been exposed to estrogen and progesterone for a longer time. Estrogen and progesterone are hormones that control the development of secondary sex characteristics, such as breast development, and pregnancy. The production of estrogen and progesterone decreases with age, with a steep decrease around menopause. Longer exposure to these hormones increases breast cancer risk.

Timing of pregnancy. Having a first pregnancy after age 35 or if you've never had a full-term pregnancy brings a higher risk of breast cancer. Pregnancy may help protect against breast cancer because it pushes breast cells into their final phase of maturation.

Hormone replacement therapy after menopause. Using hormone therapy with both estrogen and progestin after menopause, often called hormone replacement therapy, within the past 5 years or for several years increases the risk of breast cancer. In fact, the number of new breast cancers diagnosed has dropped substantially as there is now less use of postmenopausal hormone therapy. However, women who have taken only estrogen, without previously receiving progestin, for up to 5 years (because they had their uterus removed for other reasons) appear to have a slightly lower risk of breast cancer.

Oral contraceptives or birth control pills: Some studies suggest that oral contraceptives to prevent pregnancy slightly increase the risk of breast cancer, while others have shown no link between the use of oral contraceptives and development of breast cancer. Research on this topic is ongoing.

Race and ethnicity: Breast cancer is the most common cancer diagnosis in women, other than skin cancer, regardless of race. White women are more likely to develop breast cancer than Black women, but among women younger than 45, the disease is more common in Black women than in White women. Black women are also more likely to die from the disease. Reasons for survival differences may include differences in biology, other health conditions, and socioeconomic factors affecting access to medical care.

Breast density: Having dense breast tissue generally means you have more milk glands, milk ducts, and supportive tissue in the breast than fatty tissue. Dense breast tissue is a measure used to describe mammogram images as opposed to how the breast feels. Breast density usually decreases with age. Having dense breast tissue increases the risk of developing breast cancer. In addition, dense breast tissue may make it more difficult to detect a tumor on standard imaging tests, such as mammography. Some states require that mammogram results include information about breast density if the results show that a person has dense breast tissue. However, at this time, there are no special screening guidelines for people with dense breasts.

Lifestyle factors: As with other types of cancer, studies continue to show that various lifestyle factors may contribute to the development of breast cancer.

- Weight: Recent studies have shown that being post-menopausal and being overweight or obese brings an increased risk of breast cancer. There is also a higher risk of the cancer coming back after treatment.
- Physical activity: A lower amount of physical activity is associated with an increased risk of developing breast cancer and a higher risk of having the cancer come back after treatment.

- Alcohol: Current research suggests that having more than 1 to 2 servings of alcohol, including beer, wine, and spirits, per day raises the risk of breast cancer. General recommendations are typically to limit your alcohol intake to 3 to 4 servings per week.

- Food: There is no reliable research that confirms that eating or avoiding specific foods increases the risk of developing breast cancer or having the cancer come back after treatment. However, eating more fruits and vegetables and fewer animal fats is linked with many health benefits, including a slight decrease in the risk of breast cancer.

- Socioeconomic factors: More affluent women in all racial and ethnic groups have a higher risk of developing breast cancer than less affluent women in the same groups. These differences may be due to variations in diet, pregnancy factors such as age at first pregnancy and number of pregnancies, and other risk factors. Women living in poverty are more likely to be diagnosed at an advanced stage and are less likely to survive the disease than more affluent women. This is likely due to multiple factors, including lifestyle factors and other health conditions such as obesity and tumor biology. Access to health care and the availability of treatment play additional roles.

Radiation exposure at a young age: Exposure to ionizing radiation at a young age may increase a woman's risk of breast cancer.

**Prevention**

Different factors cause different types of cancer. Researchers continue to look into what factors cause breast cancer, and how to prevent it. Although there is no proven way to completely prevent breast cancer, you may be able to lower your risk.

For those at higher risk, the following options may help reduce your risk of breast cancer. Talk with your health care team for more information about your personal risk of breast cancer.

Let's look at what could help prevent this cancer.

Lifestyle choices to lower cancer risk: One way to lower your risk of breast cancer is by getting regular physical activity. Studies suggest that 30 to 60 minutes per day of moderate- to high-intensity physical activity is associated with a lower breast cancer risk. Other ways to lower your risk include staying at a healthy weight and avoiding the use of hormone replacement therapy with both estrogen and progestin after menopause. Breastfeeding may also reduce breast cancer risk. Learn about more lifestyle choices that may help lower your risk of breast cancer.

Surgery to lower cancer risk: When there is a BRCA1 or BRCA2 genetic mutation present, which substantially increases the risk of breast cancer, preventive removal of the breasts may be considered. This procedure is called a prophylactic mastectomy. It appears to reduce the risk of developing breast cancer by at least 90% to 95%. People with these genetic mutations should also consider the preventive removal of the ovaries and fallopian tubes, called a prophylactic salpingo-oophorectomy.

This procedure can reduce the risk of developing ovarian cancer, and possibly breast cancer, by stopping the ovaries from making estrogen. When considering having these procedures, it is important to talk with your doctor about possible physical and emotional side effects.

Drugs to lower cancer risk: If you have a higher than usual risk of developing breast cancer, consider talking with your doctor about drugs that may help prevent breast cancer. This approach is called "chemoprevention." For breast cancer, this is the use of hormone-blocking drugs to reduce cancer risk.

- Tamoxifen (available as a generic drug): Tamoxifen is a type of drug called a selective estrogen receptor modulator (SERM). It is often used as a treatment for breast cancer for people who already have the disease. Tamoxifen blocks the effects of estrogen on tumor growth. Tamoxifen may be an option to help lower the risk of breast cancer, specifically ER-positive breast cancer, for women who are age 35 or older. Research has shown that it may also be effective to reduce the risk of breast cancer and cause minimal side effects for women with non-invasive breast cancer (also called ductal carcinoma in situ, or DCIS) or precancerous breast conditions called LCIS or atypical hyperplasia of the breast. It is not recommended for those with a history of blood clots, stroke, or who are immobilized (unable to move around) for a long time. It is also not recommended during pregnancy or if you are trying to become pregnant, or during breastfeeding.

The side effects of tamoxifen may include hot flashes, vaginal discharge, sexual side effects, mood changes, and a higher risk of developing uterine cancer, blood clots, and stroke.

- Raloxifene (available as a generic drug): Raloxifene is also a SERM. It is often used to prevent osteoporosis (thinning of the bones) after menopause. Raloxifene may be an option after the age of 35 when there is a higher risk of breast cancer and after menopause. Raloxifene can be used for longer than 5 years and may reduce the risk of bone loss in addition to lowering breast cancer risk. It is not recommended for women who have not been through menopause or who have a history of blood clots, stroke, or are immobilized for a long time. The side effects of raloxifene may include hot flashes, leg cramps, swelling of the legs and arms, weight gain, stroke, blood clots, vaginal dryness, and pain during sexual intercourse. Women taking raloxifene are less likely to develop blood clots, uterine problems, and cataracts than people taking tamoxifen.

- Aromatase inhibitors (AIs): AIs reduce the amount of estrogen in the body by blocking estrogen production. There are 3 AIs that may be options for lowering breast cancer risk after menopause when there is a higher risk of developing breast cancer: exemestane (Aromasin), anastrozole (Arimidex), and letrozole (Femara). While they are only approved by the U.S. Food and Drug Administration

(FDA) for use in breast cancer treatment and not in the risk-reduction setting, large, randomized clinical trials have shown that these drugs are effective in reducing the risk of developing breast cancer. Talk with your doctor about whether an AI might be right for you. AIs can be used as an alternative to tamoxifen for women who have a higher risk of breast cancer and who have been through menopause. AIs are not used to treat women who have not been through menopause and are not usually recommended for those with osteoporosis.

The side effects of AIs may include hot flashes, fatigue, difficulty sleeping, diarrhea, joint and muscle pain, vaginal dryness, and bone loss.

# Chapter 2: Diagnosis and Medical Team

## 2.1 The Diagnosis Process

There are so many tests and procedures used to diagnose breast cancer.

Breast exam: Your doctor will check both of your breasts and lymph nodes in your armpit, feeling for any lumps or other abnormalities.

Mammogram: A mammogram is an X-ray of the breast. Mammograms are commonly used to screen for breast cancer. If an abnormality is detected on a screening mammogram, your doctor may recommend a diagnostic mammogram to further evaluate that abnormality.

Breast ultrasound: Ultrasound uses sound waves to produce images of structures deep within the body. Ultrasound may be used to determine whether a new breast lump is a solid mass or a fluid-filled cyst.

Removing a sample of breast cells for testing (biopsy): A biopsy is the only definitive way to make a diagnosis of breast cancer. During a biopsy, your doctor uses a specialized needle device guided by X-ray or another imaging test to extract a core of tissue from the suspicious area. Often, a small metal marker is left at the site within your breast so the area can be easily identified on future imaging tests.

Biopsy samples are sent to a laboratory for analysis where experts determine whether the cells are cancerous. A biopsy sample is also analyzed to determine the type of cells involved in breast cancer, the aggressiveness (grade) of the cancer, and whether the cancer cells have hormone receptors or other receptors that may influence your treatment options.

Breast magnetic resonance imaging (MRI): An MRI machine uses a magnet and radio waves to create pictures of the interior of your breast. Before a breast MRI, you receive an injection of dye. Unlike other types of imaging tests, an MRI doesn't use radiation to create the images.

## 2.2 Assembling Your Medical Team

Receiving a breast cancer diagnosis can be overwhelming and emotionally challenging. One of the most critical steps you can take after diagnosis is to assemble a skilled and compassionate medical team to guide you through your breast cancer journey. Your medical team will play a central role in developing your treatment plan, providing support, and helping you make informed decisions. Here's a closer look at how to assemble your medical team:

Breast Surgeon: A breast surgeon specializes in the surgical treatment of breast cancer. They are responsible for performing biopsies, lumpectomies, mastectomies, and lymph node removal if necessary. Your breast surgeon will be a key member of your team.

Oncologist: Medical oncologists specialize in treating cancer with medications, including chemotherapy, hormone therapy, targeted therapy, and immunotherapy. Depending on your treatment plan, you may work closely with a medical oncologist.

Radiation Oncologist: If radiation therapy is part of your treatment plan, a radiation oncologist will administer this treatment. They specialize in using high-energy rays to target and destroy cancer cells while minimizing damage to healthy tissue.

Pathologist: Pathologists are experts in diagnosing diseases by examining tissue samples. They play a crucial role in confirming your breast cancer diagnosis and providing information about the type and stage of cancer.

Radiologist: Radiologists are responsible for interpreting imaging tests such as mammograms, ultrasounds, and MRIs. They help identify the size and location of tumors and assess the extent of cancer's spread.

Nurse Navigator: Nurse navigators are valuable members of your team who provide support and guidance throughout your treatment. They help coordinate appointments, explain medical terminology, and connect you with resources and support services.

Genetic Counselor: If you have a family history of breast cancer or carry specific genetic mutations, a genetic counselor can help you understand your risk and make informed decisions about genetic testing and preventive measures.

Supportive Care Specialists: Depending on your needs, your medical team may include social workers, psychologists, nutritionists, and physical therapists who provide support and address the emotional and practical aspects of your care.

Primary Care Physician: Your primary care physician remains an essential part of your medical team. They can help coordinate your overall health and well-being, manage any pre-existing conditions, and monitor your general health during and after treatment.

Second Opinions: Seeking a second opinion from another medical professional can provide additional perspective on your diagnosis and treatment options. Many healthcare providers encourage second opinions as part of the decision-making process.

# Chapter 3: Treatment Options

## 3.1 Surgery: Lumpectomy VS Mastectomy

Before I get into the advantages and disadvantages of each type of breast cancer surgery, let's quickly define the two procedures and touch on what might make one option more appropriate than another for some women.

Lumpectomy surgery (also called breast-conserving surgery) removes only the tumor and a margin of surrounding healthy tissue (and often one or more lymph nodes in the armpit).

Mastectomy is a surgery to remove the entire breast (and often some lymph nodes in the armpit).

While any breast cancer patient can choose to undergo a mastectomy, only some are candidates for a lumpectomy. For early-stage breast cancer, if the tumor is small enough for a lumpectomy followed by radiation therapy, the two procedures typically have similar overall survival rates, although lumpectomy followed by radiation therapy has a slightly higher rate of recurrence. The risk of cancer metastasizing (or spreading to other parts of the body) is about the same with either surgery.

Recent advances in surgical techniques and pre-surgical cancer treatments (such as immunotherapy or targeted therapy) allow the breast surgeon to spare more healthy tissue, meaning more women are able to undergo the less invasive option of a lumpectomy.

This book isn't the best venue for a thorough discussion of the decision-making factors that determine who's a good fit for a lumpectomy, because those conversations largely rely on individual considerations unique to each patient. But we can share these two basic factors that tend to rule out a lumpectomy.

- The patient can't undergo radiation therapy if a woman is pregnant or has other medical conditions that may predispose her to experiencing severe side effects from radiation therapy, she wouldn't be able to undergo a lumpectomy, because, to lower the risk of recurrence, a lumpectomy is almost always followed by radiation therapy to destroy remaining cancer cells.

- Also, if The tumor is too large compared to the size of the breast then the decision may also depend on the location and type of tumor. Sometimes a small tumor is located in a part of the breast that makes it difficult to conserve much breast tissue, so a lumpectomy isn't a viable option.

Now let's dive into the advantages and disadvantages of Mastectomy.

For some women, removing the entire breast provides greater peace of mind (just get the whole thing out of there!). Radiation therapy may still be needed, depending on the results of the pathology.

Mastectomy has some possible disadvantages:

- Mastectomy takes longer and is more extensive than lumpectomy, with more post-surgery side effects and a longer recuperation time.
- It means a permanent loss of your breast.
- You are likely to have additional surgeries to reconstruct your breast after mastectomy.

Let's look out the advantages and disadvantages of Lumpectomy.

The main advantage of lumpectomy is that it can preserve much of the appearance and sensation of your breast. It is a less invasive surgery, so your recovery time is shorter and easier than with mastectomy.

Lumpectomy has a few potential disadvantages:

- You are likely to have 5 to 7 weeks of radiation therapy, 5 days per week, after lumpectomy surgery to make sure the cancer is gone.

- Radiation therapy may affect the timing of reconstruction and possibly your reconstruction options after surgery. Radiation therapy also may affect your options for later surgery to lift or balance your breasts.

- There is a somewhat higher risk of developing a local recurrence of the cancer after lumpectomy than after mastectomy. However, local recurrence can be treated successfully with mastectomy.

- The breast cannot safely tolerate additional radiation if there is a recurrence in the same breast after lumpectomy. This is true for either a recurrence of the same cancer, or for a new cancer. If you have a second cancer in the same breast, your doctor will usually recommend that you have a mastectomy.

- You may need to have one or more additional surgeries after your initial lumpectomy. During lumpectomy, the surgeon removes the cancer tumor and some of the normal tissue around it (called the margins). A pathologist looks to see if cancer cells are in the margins. If there are cancer cells, more tissue needs to be removed until the margins are free of cancer. Ideally, this is all done during the lumpectomy, but analyzing the margins can take about a week. So sometimes after the pathology report is done, the margins are found to contain cancer cells and more surgery (called a re-excision) is needed.

## 3.2 Radiation Therapy

Radiation therapy for breast cancer uses high-energy X-rays, protons or other particles to kill cancer cells. Rapidly growing cells, such as cancer cells, are more susceptible to the effects of radiation therapy than are normal cells.

The X-rays or particles are painless and invisible. You are not radioactive after treatment, so it is safe to be around other people, including children.

Radiation therapy for breast cancer may be delivered through:

External radiation: A machine delivers radiation from outside your body to the breast. This is the most common type of radiation therapy used for breast cancer.

Internal radiation (brachytherapy): After you have surgery to remove the cancer, your doctor temporarily places a radiation-delivery device in your breast in the area where the cancer once was. A radioactive source is placed into the device for short periods of time over the course of your treatment.

Radiation therapy may be used to treat breast cancer at almost every stage. Radiation therapy is an effective way to reduce your risk of breast cancer recurring after surgery. In addition, it is commonly used to ease the symptoms caused by cancer that has spread to other parts of the body (metastatic breast cancer).

### 3.3 Chemotherapy

Chemotherapy for breast cancer uses drugs to target and destroy breast cancer cells. These drugs are usually injected directly into a vein through a needle or taken by mouth as pills.

It is frequently used in addition to other treatments, such as surgery, radiation or hormone therapy. Chemotherapy can be used to increase the chance of a cure, decrease the risk of the cancer returning, alleviate symptoms from the cancer or help people with cancer live longer with a better quality of life.

If the cancer has recurred or spread, chemotherapy may control the breast cancer to help you live longer. Or it can help ease symptoms the cancer is causing.

It also carries a risk of side effects — some temporary and mild, others more serious or permanent. Your doctor can help you decide whether chemotherapy for breast cancer is a good choice for you.

## 3.4 Hormone Therapy

Hormone therapy is only used for breast cancers that are found to have receptors for the naturally occurring hormones estrogen or progesterone.

It is often used after surgery to reduce the risk that the cancer might return. Hormone therapy also may be used to shrink a cancer before surgery. If the cancer shrinks, it may be possible to remove less breast tissue during surgery. Using hormone therapy before surgery also gives your health care team information about how well your cancer responds to this treatment.

If your cancer has spread to other parts of your body, hormone therapy for breast cancer may help control it.

**3.5 Targeted Therapy**

Targeted drug therapy uses medicines that are directed at (target) proteins on breast cancer cells that help them grow, spread, and live longer. Targeted drugs work to destroy cancer cells or slow down their growth. They have side effects different from chemotherapy.

Some targeted therapy drugs, for example, monoclonal antibodies, work in more than one way to control cancer cells and may also be considered immunotherapy because they boost the immune system.

Like chemotherapy, these drugs enter the bloodstream and reach almost all areas of the body, which makes them useful against cancers that have spread to distant parts of the body. Targeted drugs sometimes work even when chemo drugs do not. Some targeted drugs can help other types of treatment work better.

## 3.6 Immunotherapy

Immunotherapy is the use of medicines to boost a person's own immune system to recognize and destroy cancer cells more effectively. Immunotherapy typically works on specific proteins involved in the immune system to enhance the immune response. These drugs have side effects different from those of chemotherapy.

Some immunotherapy drugs, for example, monoclonal antibodies, work in more than one way to control cancer cells and may also be considered targeted therapy because they block a specific protein on the cancer cell to keep it from growing.

# Chapter 4: Navigating Treatment

## 4.1 Coping with Side Effects

Breast cancer treatments come in a variety of forms and combinations. Your medical team will take different factors into account when deciding how to best treat your particular form of cancer.

Each type of cancer treatment can have side effects, but it's important to remember that not everyone experiences them, and not all of them will affect you or your loved one.

Side effects can be short or long-term, but are usually temporary and stop when treatment finishes. If you are experiencing severe side effects, it's important to talk to your medical team. Treatments are available to relieve common side effects, and many patients find self-care treatments extremely helpful.

For chemotherapy, side effects can include hair loss, blood changes and blood clots, sickness and digestive problems, sore mouth, fatigue, changes to skin and nails, and fertility problems.

For radiation therapy, many side effects are similar to those of chemotherapy - such as sore skin, hair loss in the area of treatment, sore throat and mouth, nausea, fatigue and fertility issues.

Some people develop lymphoedema as a side effect of radiation therapy too. It is a condition causing a build-up of fluid in the body's tissues, which can happen when the lymphatic system is damaged through radiation therapy.

Hormone therapy, the side effects of hormone therapy can include fatigue, nausea and joint and muscle pain. Women can experience menopausal symptoms, hot flashes and vaginal dryness or discharge, and men can suffer from impotence.

Surgery, side effects of breast cancer surgery can include bleeding, infection, pain, swelling and the formation of hard scar tissue.

It can be difficult to cope with the physical changes of breast cancer surgery. Reconstructive surgery, specialist breast-shaped prosthesis and underwear can help restore your confidence, but it's important to get support for the emotional ups and downs of the procedure and its after-effects

Targeted Therapy, side effects may include fever, tiredness, joint aches, nausea, headaches, itchy eyes with or without blurred vision, diarrhea, bleeding and bruising, and high blood pressure. Less commonly, some targeted therapy drugs can affect the way the heart, thyroid, liver or lungs work, or increase the risk of getting an infection. If left untreated, some side effects can become serious.

Immunotherapy, some common side effects are diarrhea, organ inflammation, infection, fatigue, etc

Coping with these side effects can be challenging at times but I can assure you a physical self care can be of help and soothe your body and mind. Try using topical creams for sensitive skin, ice lollies for sore mouths, and beautiful hats and headscarves to help manage hair loss.

Building a support network will help you and those around you. Talking through the procedures openly can reduce strain on relationships and help everyone share the emotional load.

Joining breast cancer support groups to talk through shared experiences can help you realise you are not alone and provide a vital system of peer support.

Complementary therapies such as acupuncture, reflexology and massage can help you relax and calm your nervous system, reducing stress and anxiety.

Gentle exercise, such as yoga and walking, can boost your physical and mental wellbeing by giving your mind a focus and supporting your physical recovery.

## 4.2 Emotional and Psychological Support

Healthcare professionals may recommend both group and individual therapy to help manage stress or depression for people with cancer.

Ask your breast cancer care team or a social worker to refer you to a licensed psychologist, psychiatrist, or mental health counselor.

These professionals may use an approach known as cognitive behavioral therapy. They can also prescribe medications if they think you'd benefit from an approach that involves more than one method.

Due to the COVID-19 pandemic, many of these services have transitioned to virtual sessions. This is great news for anyone living in a rural area who may have trouble finding a local therapist who specializes in mental health for people with cancer.

These virtual sessions are sometimes called teletherapy. You can receive teletherapy through video chat, phone calls, and even text messaging.

## 4.3 Managing Pain and Discomfort

Once an assessment of your pain has been completed, a management plan can be developed. This is an agreed outcome of discussions between you and your treating team. Pain management plans include a holistic approach to ensure that the plan addresses your physical, emotional and social needs.

Your pain management plan may include:

- The use of medication such as analgesics (painkillers).
- Physiotherapy to treat the specific parts of your body that are affected by pain.
- Exercise plan – exercise has been shown to be very effective in treating chronic pain. An exercise physiologist or physiotherapist can tailor an exercise program to your needs.

## 4.4 Complementary Therapies

Many people use complementary therapies, such as acupuncture and prayer, during or after their breast cancer care. You may also hear the terms integrative therapies or complementary health approaches.

Complementary therapies may relieve some side effects and improve quality of life. They do not treat breast cancer.

Some complementary therapies can interfere with breast cancer treatment. To avoid problems, talk with your health care provider about possible benefits and risks before you use complementary therapy.

# Chapter 5: Life During Treatment

## 5.1 Balancing Work and Treatment

The impact of a breast cancer diagnosis on work life varies from person to person. For some, the effect is minimal. For others, there might be some questions about how to manage work and treatment. You may have an understanding supervisor, a flexible schedule, and an encouraging team to support you through treatment. For others, there might be some questions about how to manage work and treatment: What do I tell my boss? Should I take time off from work for treatment? How will I pay the bills?

Here are some strategies for managing the emotional, physical, and legal aspects of balancing your job and your breast cancer treatment.

First, tell your boss and co-workers about your breast cancer diagnosis. The first question you may ask yourself when thinking about talking to your boss or co-workers about your breast cancer diagnosis is, "Should I tell them?" You don't have to tell anyone at work, unless it is apparent that your diagnosis or treatment will interfere with your work schedule or your ability to do your job. Keep in mind that if you decide not to discuss your health at work, some questions may be raised if your productivity is affected or if you need to take a lot of time off because of treatment appointments.

You might decide to just tell some people — your supervisor, your closest colleagues, or someone with whom you share responsibilities.

Or you could decide to tell everyone, depending on how comfortable you feel. Keep in mind that people may react differently; you may receive support from some co-workers, while others might not be as comfortable with the conversation.

Second, let your doctor know if you'll be able to work during your treatments so he/she may be able to schedule your treatments around your working hours or suggest ways to manage work stress while you're in treatment. You also can ask your doctor if any of your treatments have side effects that could affect your daily routine, such as nausea and fatigue.

Third, take time off from work for treatment if you feel you won't be able to cope with the stress to avoid further complications.

## 5.2 Nutrition and Diet

If you're recovering from surgery, receiving chemotherapy or radiation, or having other breast cancer treatment, your main focus is on getting rid of the cancer. Eating well will help you stay strong by giving your body the nutrients it needs.

You and your doctor can't predict exactly how your treatment will affect you. Your general health and weight before your diagnosis play a role. So do the type, amount, and length of treatment you are receiving. As you move through your treatment, listen to your body and respond to what it needs. You may continue to enjoy cooking and eating and have a normal appetite. Or you might have days when you don't feel like eating anything, days when you want to eat everything, and times when only some things taste good. It's best to have a flexible, healthy eating plan to help you deal with your body's changing needs and wants.

A healthy diet — one with a variety of foods that includes lots of fruits and vegetables and regular protein — gives you the reserves of nutrients you need to keep your strength up while you're being treated for breast cancer. These reserves also help rebuild your body's tissues and keep your immune system strong to help fight off infection. Plus, a healthy diet can help you manage treatment side effects. There is evidence that some cancer treatments actually work better in people who are eating enough calories and protein. While you're having breast cancer treatment, it's more important than ever that you eat a healthy diet.

## 5.3 Exercise and Physical Activity

Exercise and physical activity are integral parts of breast cancer treatment that have many benefits for people with cancer. They can reduce fatigue and improve cardiovascular fitness, strength, balance, and overall confidence and emotional well-being. For people with breast cancer, exercise is typically safe to continue throughout treatment, including during chemotherapy, radiation therapy, and surgery. However, certain exercises may require modification based on your fatigue levels, and different precautions may need to be taken at different phases of your treatment plan.

It is important to remember that each person with breast cancer is unique, and your personal tolerance for movement during breast cancer treatment may vary. Always talk with your health care team if you have any questions or concerns about exercising during treatment. Your health care team can refer you to a physical therapist or trained breast cancer exercise specialist who can tailor your exercise program to meet your specific needs and goals.

## 5.4 Family and Relationships

Family and relationships are the cornerstone of our lives, shaping our sense of belonging, identity, and emotional well-being. They provide us with a support system, a source of love, and a foundation upon which we build our lives. Nurturing healthy family relationships is vital for our overall happiness and mental health. A good family and relationships will offer emotional support during this challenging time of cancer treatment.

Also, it gives a sense of belonging and identity by reminding us who we are and where we come from.

It reduces stress and promotes mental wellbeing as well as personal growth.

# Chapter 6: After Treatment: Survivorship

## 6.1 Life Beyond Treatment

Your appearance might be affected by breast cancer and its treatments, like scars from surgery, or hair loss from chemotherapy. These changes may affect your body image and self-esteem.

Getting used to the changes will take some time, but research has shown that the sooner you accept the changes, the easier you will find it to gain confidence in your appearance. You might be shocked or unhappy the first few times you see yourself in the mirror, but these feelings will lessen over time as you get used to your appearance. Prosthesis or reconstruction is an option to restore your natural appearance after breast cancer surgery and may help you feel more confident. The choice for a prosthesis or reconstruction is yours, and it is okay if you do not want to receive either.

If you had surgery for breast cancer, you will have to consider the type of bra you wear during the first year after your surgery. Bras with soft seams, a wide underband, full cups, adjustable straps, and no wires will be more comfortable. The needs for your bra may change depending on your weight or other treatment-related changes. Immediately after surgery, you are likely to prefer a bra that is loose, due to the swelling you will experience.

Breast cancer treatment can also cause menopausal symptoms, and you might find these manageable or difficult to cope with. If you have already been through menopause, you may still re-experience menopausal symptoms. Treatments that can cause menopausal symptoms include hormone therapies, ovarian suppression, and chemotherapy.

If you are concerned with any of the symptoms you experience, you should talk to your treatment team.

Learning to live with breast cancer comes with stress and worries, but you are not alone in this journey and your healthcare team will always have your back. For some women with breast cancer, their cancer may never go away completely and might require continuous treatments to keep it under control. Your doctor will arrange regular follow-ups to monitor your condition while supporting you to adapt and live with any side effects of your treatment. You can also discuss with your doctor regarding concerns with whether the cancer will return, and if it does, what are your options. Treatment will depend on where it comes back, and what treatments you have already had before

## 6.2 Follow Up Care and Monitoring

Many women are relieved to be finished with breast cancer treatment, but also worry about the cancer coming back and can feel lost when they don't see their cancer care team as often.

But for some women with advanced breast cancer, the cancer may never go away completely. These women may continue to get treatments to help keep the breast cancer under control and to help relieve symptoms from it.

Learning to live with advanced breast cancer that doesn't go away can have its own types of stress and uncertainty.

Even if you have completed breast cancer treatment, your doctors still will want to watch you closely, so it's very important for you to go to all of your follow-up appointments. During these visits, your doctors will ask if you are having any problems and will examine you. Lab tests and imaging tests typically aren't needed after treatment for most early-stage breast cancers. But they might be done in some women who are having symptoms to see if they're the result of the cancer returning or are from treatment-related side effects.

Almost any cancer treatment can have side effects. Some might only last for a few days or weeks, but others might last a long time. Some side effects might not even show up until years after you have finished treatment. Your doctor visits are a good time for you to ask questions and talk about any changes or problems you notice or concerns you have. However, if concerns about your cancer come up between visits, you shouldn't wait until your next scheduled visit. Call your doctor's office right away.

**Typical follow-up schedules**

Your follow-up schedule can depend on many factors, including the type of breast cancer, how advanced it was when it was found (the stage of the cancer), and how it was (or is being) treated.

Doctor visits: If you have finished treatment, your follow-up visits will probably be every few months at first. The longer you have been free of cancer, the less often the appointments are needed. After 5 years, they are typically done about once a year.

Mammograms: If you had breast-conserving surgery (lumpectomy or partial mastectomy), you will probably have a mammogram about 6 to 12 months after surgery and radiation are completed, and then at least every year after that. Women who've had a mastectomy (removal of the entire breast) typically no longer need mammograms on that side. But unless you've had both breasts removed, you still need to have yearly mammograms on the remaining breast. To learn more, see Mammograms After Breast Cancer Surgery.

Pelvic exams: If you are taking either of the hormone drugs tamoxifen or toremifene and still have your uterus, your doctor will likely recommend pelvic exams every year because these drugs can increase your risk of uterine (endometrial) cancer. This risk is highest in women who have gone through menopause. Be sure to tell your doctor right away about any unusual vaginal bleeding, such as bleeding or spotting after menopause, bleeding or spotting between periods, or a change in your periods. Although this is usually caused by something that isn't cancer, it can also be the first sign of uterine cancer.

Bone density tests: If you are taking a hormone drug called an aromatase inhibitor (such as anastrozole, letrozole, or exemestane) for early-stage breast cancer, or if treatment puts you into menopause, your doctor will want to monitor your bone health and may consider testing your bone density.

Other tests: Other tests such as blood tests and imaging tests (like bone scans, x-rays, or CT or PET scans) are not a standard part of follow-up for most women who've been treated for breast cancer, because they haven't been shown to help them live longer. But one or more of these tests might be done if you have symptoms or physical exam findings that suggest that the cancer might have come back.

If symptoms, exams, or tests suggest your cancer might have returned, imaging tests such as an x-ray, CT scan, PET scan, MRI scan, bone scan, and/or a biopsy may be done.

## 6.3 Embracing Your Survivorship

You've reached a milestone in your breast cancer care. Active treatment to get rid of the cancer is done. Maybe you even "rang the bell" with family, friends, and your medical team looking on to celebrate your big moment.

Depending on your diagnosis and choices, you may have soldiered through treatment like surgery, radiation, and chemotherapy. No doubt you're relieved, but maybe a bit nervous, too. "Now what?" you may ask. "Am I a breast cancer survivor? Could it rear its ugly head again?" That's a question that lives in your head 24/7.

The exciting news is that most women successfully treated for early breast cancer will be done with it for good. But that's not everyone, and the definition of "survivorship" means different things to different people.

One way to regain a sense of control is to take steps that improve your quality of life after breast cancer treatment. If you haven't made healthy lifestyle changes already, now's the time to start:

*Exercise. Ask your doctor how much you can do. In cancer survivors, exercise can:

-Prevent it from coming back

-Help with fatigue and pain from previous treatment or your current medications

-Improve your mood and sleep

Those are just a few of the benefits of moving. Start slowly, but try to work up to at least half an hour a day, 5 days a week.

*Keep a healthy weight. You may have lost or gained weight during breast cancer treatment. If you need help to get to a healthy weight, talk to your doctor. Nausea or pain can affect your ability to eat. Your care team may refer you to a registered dietitian who can help you tip the scales in your favor.

*Stop smoking. Lighting up can pave the way for recurrence or increase your chances of getting another type of cancer. Plus, quitting improves your overall health. Talk to your doctor if you're having trouble stopping.

*Limit alcohol. Talk to your doctor about what's safe for you. Some doctors say no more than two drinks a week, while others say cut out booze altogether.

# Chapter 7: Supporting Loved ones

## 7.1 Communicating With Families and Friends

As you go through treatment your needs will change. You may have some weeks where you need more help than others. Communicating that to family and friends is key. Some things might be hard or awkward to discuss, but it's better to bring them up sooner rather than later, before they become bigger issues.

Here are a few common topics for you to keep an open dialogue about:

Changing responsibilities and how to adjust to new family roles when it comes to daily tasks, chores, errands, events, and activities.

Setting the right expectations for what everyone is able to do given their personal needs, mental state, and physical limitations.

Money matters, including how to pay for potential medical costs and living expenses.

Thoughts about your next steps for medical care: It could be that you and your partner have different opinions. It's good for you to listen to each other.

Feelings: At different times, you or your loved ones may feel overwhelmed, anxious, or depressed. Keep tabs on how each other is doing and talk through things.

At first, you may find it difficult to talk about these things, but over time, it will get easier. It will help you get the support you need, and it will help them to know how best to help.
You or your loved ones may say or do the wrong thing sometimes, but keep in mind, everyone is on the same team. Be patient with each other as you learn how to navigate your new roles and life together.

## 7.2 Helping Children Understand

For many young mothers, one of the first reactions to being diagnosed with breast cancer is "What about my kids?" There isn't one right way to help children cope, but here are some helpful guidelines you can follow:

Communication is key: Children of all ages tend to be good at picking up parents' distress, even when parents think they are hiding it well. Let them know they are not to blame for your worries so they don't make up their own explanations for what's wrong.

Use the word cancer: A problem with using words like "sick" or "boo-boo" is that children hear these words applied to themselves when they have colds or scrapes. They can feel confused when you don't recover as quickly as they do and may worry that getting sick will be just as hard for them the next time.

Let children know they did not cause nor can they catch cancer. This alleviates children making up reasons.

Tell them what to expect during treatment and how it will affect their day-to-day lives. Tell them, for example, who will care for them while you are at treatment.

Tell children about your prognosis: Use language to match with your child's age/developmental understanding. Have other family members, clergy or a therapist present for these conversations to relieve some of the burden and provide support. Consider making teachers and/or a school counselor/social worker aware of your diagnosis.

Keep lines of communication open, and check in often.

## 7.3 Caregiver Support

A breast cancer diagnosis can be an overwhelming and challenging experience, not only for the person diagnosed but also for their loved ones. As a family caregiver, your role is crucial in providing emotional support, helping with practical matters, and being a source of strength throughout this journey.

Here are some tips to support a loved one with breast cancer:

Educate Yourself: The first step in becoming an effective caregiver is to educate yourself about breast cancer. Understand the type and stage of your loved one's cancer, treatment options, and potential side effects. This knowledge will enable you to have informed discussions with healthcare providers and provide better emotional support.

Be a Good Listener: Listening is one of the most powerful ways to support your loved one. Allow them to express their fears, concerns, and emotions without judgment. Sometimes, simply lending an empathetic ear can provide immense comfort.

Attend Medical Appointments: Accompany your loved one to medical appointments if they are comfortable with it. Taking notes during these visits can help your loved one remember important information and questions to ask. This also demonstrates your commitment to their care.

Offer Practical Help: Breast cancer treatment often comes with physical challenges. Offer practical assistance with daily tasks like cooking, cleaning, and transportation to medical appointments. Additionally, consider helping with research on treatment options, insurance, and financial resources.

Encourage Self-Care: Remind your loved one to prioritize self-care. Encourage them to maintain a healthy diet, exercise, and get enough rest. Supporting their well-being can contribute to their overall strength and resilience during treatment.

Emotional Support: Breast cancer can bring about a rollercoaster of emotions. Be patient, understanding, and empathetic. Offer a shoulder to cry on, but also encourage positive thinking and hope. Sometimes, a heartfelt note or a small gesture of kindness can brighten their day.

Respect Their Choices: Every individual's breast cancer journey is unique.

Respect your loved one's choices when it comes to their treatment plan, even if they differ from what you might have in mind. They should feel in control of their decisions and treatment.

Help Manage Side Effects: Chemotherapy, radiation, and surgery can come with various side effects. Be prepared to assist your loved one in managing these, whether it's helping with medications, providing a comfortable space for rest, or being a calming presence during tough times.

Take Care of Yourself: Caring for a loved one with breast cancer can be emotionally and physically draining. Remember to take care of your own health and well-being. A well-rested and emotionally stable caregiver is better equipped to provide support. Friends and family can only do so much and may have conflicting schedules.

Supporting a loved one with breast cancer can be a challenging and emotionally demanding role, but it's also incredibly meaningful. Your presence, love, and support can make a world of difference in their journey toward recovery. By educating yourself, being a good listener, and offering practical help, you can be an invaluable source of strength during this difficult time. Together, you can navigate the challenges of breast cancer and emerge stronger than ever.

# Conclusion

Breast cancer is the most common type of tumor in women in most parts of the world. Although stabilized in Western countries, its incidence is increasing in other continents. Prevention of breast cancer is difficult because the causes are not well known. We know of many risk factors such as nulliparity, late age at first pregnancy, little or no breastfeeding, which, however, are linked to the historic development of human society. On the contrary, a great effort is needed to improve early detection of the tumor. Screening programs among the female population should therefore be implemented. The early discovery of a small breast carcinoma leads to a very high rate of curability and entails very mild types of treatment, with preservation of the body image. Treatments are improving, but a strict interdisciplinary approach is essential. It is conceivable that in all countries specialized centers or units for breast cancer management should be set up.

Want to learn about living with and beating prostate cancer? click here to get a copy of my book on amazon about it.

Away from this book, it would be really appreciated if you could provide a preview if you thought it was worthwhile as it would motivate me. Thanks.